How to Build Muscle and Burn Fat

By David A. Hunter

GAIN WEIGHT FAST

By DAVID A. HUNTER

<u>Obtaining the Right Mindset</u>

Before you you embark upon any kind of journey towards achieving your goals, it is important to get into the correct state of mind. You must rid yourself of any negative beliefs that can or have been hindering your progress.

Perhaps you have been accustomed to blaming bad genetics or some other misfortune that was thrown your way. I am not stating that genetics do not play a role in this at all, but until you escape from the victim mentality, you will be holding yourself back.

After you get past your self-defeating thoughts, the next step is to focus. I made my most substantial progress after I began to put my goals in front of me and just think about them all the time.

Doing this is crucial for gaining weight since you will most likely have no one else to coach you. Most people probably do not understand why you want to gain weight in the first place anyway. But obviously, it is important to you, otherwise you most likely would not be reading this.

Everybody has different reasons as to why they want to put on some weight. It could be for sports, to look healthier, or to feel healthier.

Whatever the reason may be, there is always that sense of accomplishment knowing that you took something that you believed in and went all the way with it, regardless of what anyone else thought or said.

Motivation is a must. A good way to stay inspired is to ask yourself why you want to gain weight. Constantly remind yourself how much more confident you will feel after finding success. After you set a goal and achieve it, you will build character.

The confidence gained from reaching your goal will help you down the road for the rest of your life.

From that point on, whenever you encounter an obstacle, you can simply look back and remember that what you thought was impossible is indeed possible if you just set yourself to the right state of mind.

Remind yourself of what you want to look like. You don't have to hang posters on the wall and stare at them all day, but it does help to at least have a basic idea of what you really want, and then trust yourself that you will accomplish it.

Contrary to popular belief, being underweight is really no more fun than being overweight is. So if you are ready to lose the skinny look, start thinking of yourself as you would like to be.

The next thing you need to have is persistence. The right kind of motivation will usually lead to persistence, but you have to be patient as well as careful as to not be too hard on yourself. Personally, I was thirteen years old when I decided to put on some weight. I was hoping for a lot of weight because I was pretty skinny.

Lifting weights and consuming more protein was not enough to put on much weight. I also got more sore than I should have from the workouts because I wasn't eating enough overall calories to support what I was doing.

Then I realized that I was only eating more on my workout days, but not on my days off. That was my second wake up call. I would not only require more protein and overall calories to get results, but I would also have to stay consistent.

Over the years, my weight would bounce back and forth. I would gain five pounds in a month, but lose three pounds the following week because I did not stay consistent.

Finally, I decided that enough was enough and that if I was going to get serious about gaining the weight that I needed, I would have to stay motivated enough to fuel my persistence.

As I kept myself motivated and stayed consistent, I put on about twelve pounds in just a couple of months.

The weight gain didn't stop there, it just slowed down after that. If you persist for long enough, who knows where that can take you? It will be up to you to determine how much weight you want to gain.

Just keep in mind that there is such a thing as trying to gain too much weight too fast. I know that you want it all now already, but you also need to look at the big picture and learn to see things in the long run.

The only time you should stop being consistent is if you come down with a cold, flu, or some other illness. That would be good enough reason to put your goal on hold for the time being and just shift your focus towards recovery. Just take a break and get back at it after you get well again.

This book will show you how to gain weight as soon as you can while still doing it in a healthy way.

With that said, this will be a two part book. The first will deal mostly with the nutrition side of gaining weight while the second part will talk about exercise and how to build muscle mass.

If you simply have no interest in lifting heavy weights, just stick with the nutrition part to gain weight. If you are interested in increasing muscle size then it makes sense to read the entire book all the way through.

<u>Nutrition Overlook</u>

Whether you are trying to gain muscle weight or just regular weight without putting on too much fat, nutrition should be your primary focus.

You are under your target weight because you are lacking the right kind of nutrition.

Getting enough sleep and relaxation are never bad things, but if you are not gaining the weight that you want to gain, chances are it's because you are not eating the right foods in the right quantities at the right times. You might also have trouble doing it for long enough to see any real results.

Remember that nobody is going to gain the weight for you.

It is not the same thing as learning how to drive a car. With a car, you just take the time to learn once, and then you're set. You can choose not to drive for weeks and weeks at a time and still not forget how to drive.

When it comes to a health or fitness program, you will have to continue it throughout your life. But you will grow accustomed to it once you start doing it for long enough. The food also does not need to taste bad.

I would not recommend any kind of weight gain powders or drinks. You not only wouldn't like the taste, you would also probably find them unnecessary, like I did when I was younger.

Most of that stuff is just sugar mixed with protein powder. It was like drinking wet sand as the instructions have you mix a large amount of powder with liquid. I could not find a glass big enough to put enough liquid in to match all the powder. It also costs too much money for the amount of servings that you're getting, so don't waste your time with that.

While you are learning to gain weight, I understand that you do not want to become obese either. That is why you must learn about the right kinds of food to consume so that you can start filling out your frame without gaining too much of the wrong kind of weight.

Keep in mind that it is not realistic to gain weight in a fairly short amount of time without putting on some fat. You just don't want to put on too much of it. You can always go back later on to trim off any excess fat that you are unhappy about by switching things around a bit.

For now, I would just stay focused on putting on the weight, otherwise you will just complicate things and set a roadblock on the path to your weight gain goals.

It is still alright to eat vegetables, even though they are low in calories, because you still need the vitamins and minerals they provide. I am just saying that you must emphasize the core foods that you should be eating to gain weight as I will explain later.

To start out, you should familiarize yourself with some basic nutrients which can be known as carbohydrates, protein, and fat.

It is necessary to understand the difference between these three nutrients to make sure that you are gaining the right kind of weight and not the unhealthy kind.

As I stated earlier, it is not realistic to gain much weight in a fairly short amount of time without adding on some fat. You just want to balance out these nutrients to ensure that you are minimizing the fat gains as much as you can.

Carbohydrates are used by the body for energy. It is important to have enough carbohydrates each day, especially if you are working out, as you will burn a lot of these while you are in the gym.

Carbohydrates can come in either a complex or simple form. Although both of these forms can be used for energy, there is still a difference between them as well.

Simple carbohydrates are basically certain types of sugar that are fast acting but not long lasting. A good time to consume these would be first thing in the morning when you get up, and after a workout.

Since you are not eating while you sleep, you will go into a type of starvation mode by the time you get up.

The same kind of depletion of energy can also happen during an intense workout, so it is important to consume some form of simple carbohydrate at these times to become stable again. It is usually easier to digest simple carbohydrates in liquid form.

My favorite was always grape juice, although other examples include any kind of fruit juice, fresh or frozen fruit, cookies, and candy.

It makes sense to stick to the healthier ones, though.

Complex carbohydrates are longer lasting and can be consumed all through the day. These are things you would want to have before a workout to make sure you have enough energy to perform the exercises.

Complex carbohydrates are better for gaining weight than the simple carbohydrates are, since they are generally more filling. A few examples of complex carbohydrates would be pasta, rice, and potatoes.

Protein is particularly important if you plan to build muscle mass. Regardless of whether you exercise regularly or not, you will need to consume more protein if you do not want the majority of your weight gain to be from fat.

One of the mistakes I made at the beginning of my weight gain quest was eating too many carbohydrates along with too much fat and not enough protein. Instead of getting bigger, I felt like I was starting to get fat. You should try to include some kind of protein in each one of your meals. Waffles, syrup, and bacon for breakfast would be almost all carbohydrates and fat.

Replace the waffle with a bagel, the syrup with olive oil, and the bacon with eggs, and then you have a much better meal with approximately the same amount of calories.

Good sources of protein include chicken, red meat, fish, eggs, and milk. In this case, since you want to gain weight, it would be better to stick with red meat, whole eggs, and whole milk as often as you can unless you have a cholesterol problem, in which case you should speak to your doctor first.

Fats are more highly concentrated, giving you 9 calories per gram instead of 4 calories per gram like carbohydrates and protein do.

This makes it easier to gain weight if you incorporate more fat into your diet, since you can add olive oil to many of your food choices for easy extra calories.

However, I remember getting some bad stomach pain from consuming too much cooking oil on top of all the other fatty foods that I was eating. I would not recommend more than 4 tablespoons a day.

It is good to know the difference between saturated and unsaturated fats. Saturated fats have a larger presence in butter, pork, beef, and just about all fatty meats in general.

Unsaturated fats are found in sesame seeds, corn oil, sunflower seeds, fish,soybeans, olive oil, peanuts, pumpkin seeds, walnuts, and canola oil.

Trans fats are another type of fat that you need to be aware of. This is the most unhealthy of all the fats, and it should be avoided. These fatty acids have been known to be unhealthy. Fortunately, most food products these days show you how much trans fat content is in them if you look at the back of the box.

Generally, you will want the bulk of your weight gain diet to come from whole grain complex carbohydrates, high quality protein, and healthy fats such as olive oil. Too many refined carbohydrates along with too much trans fat in your diet will possibly lead to problems down the road.

Don't Neglect Water

When you are trying to gain weight, it might sound like a waste of time to drink pure water since it does not contain any calories whatsoever.

A friend I had in school would wonder why I always had a water bottle with me at lunch. He thought that I should have been drinking nothing except milkshakes or anything else that has calories in it.

Drinking enough water when you are trying to gain weight is just as crucial as with any other scenario.

I noticed that the more food I consumed, the more water I craved. This is even more so when you are eating a lot of food that contains high amounts of sodium.

One way of making certain types of food taste better is to add a little bit of salt to them. From that alone, you will already need to boost your water intake. I have always liked adding some sea salt to baked potatoes as well as chicken.

The more obvious reasons for more water would be to meet the demands of an intense workout, or in high temperature climate conditions.

But there are other processes that many people do not consider. One of them is breathing.

Moisture is drawn out from the inside every time you exhale.

Now it is time to consider how much water you really need. The standard rule has been 8 glasses a day.

Personally, I only drink that much water occasionally, such as when I have had a lot of salt, or on a particularly hot summer day. The reason for this is because it is also bad to drink too much water. Remember that a lot of water can be taxing on the kidneys, so you should try to drink only what you need.

Finding a happy medium in this case will vary from person to person as it will depend on your sodium intake, workout intensity, and climate conditions.

A good tip is to judge by your urine color. If it is clear, you are probably overloading yourself. If it is dark yellow, then you are not drinking enough. You will want to look for a light yellow color and of course, judge by your thirst levels.

I always drink water when I crave it, even if I feel that I already had plenty. I have always believed in listening to my body, and if I feel like I need water, I always drink it as soon as I can.

Whether or not you choose to drink water during, right before, or immediately after meals should be a matter of personal preference.

Drinking water during a meal will obviously dilute it, while drinking right before or after a meal might lead to bloating.

You might feel full faster if you drink water during or anywhere around meals, so you might want to hold off on it until at least an hour before or an hour after a meal. Since you want to gain weight, it will not help you to feel full from water before you get enough calories into your system.

Depending on where you live, you may also want to get some sort of water filter that will remove contaminants from the tap water.

The chlorine found in tap water might kill bacteria, but what will you now do about the chlorine? There will also be lead as well as all sorts of other things, so take the time to invest in a quality water purification system which can be as simple as a water filter pitcher.

Just don't forget that you must change the filters regularly, depending on how much water you use.

<u>Count Your Calories</u>

Tracking your calories will be a requirement when you are trying to gain weight. Along with eating the right types of foods, this is what will make it easy to make sure that you are not putting on too much fat.

This will not be difficult since many of the food products in grocery stores have the caloric content on the back of the label.

First, you will need to know how many calories you require just to maintain your current body weight.

Start by counting how many calories you consume just to stay stuck at your current body weight. Now just add an extra 500 calories per day to your diet until you start gaining about 1 pound per week. Gaining a couple of pounds per week is not uncommon when you are following a weight gain program, but I would not go higher than this.

Putting on 1 to 2 pounds a week could add up to 4 to 8 pounds a month. That is real progress that can continue month after month. However, at some point along the way you might notice that your gains have stopped and your body weight has been the same for a couple of weeks now. An additional 500 calories a week will now be required in order to start gaining again.

I was able to consistently gain 12 pounds this way before having to add another 500 calories. Either way, at some point, your weight gain will stop, and that is when you will simply need to add even more calories until you reach the body weight that you desire.

Whether you gain 4 pounds a month or 8 pounds a month will depend on how high your activity levels are, and how fast your metabolism is. Your metabolism slows down overnight when you are not eating, so always make sure that you capitalize on this by eating before you go to bed.

I didn't have much luck with those calorie calculators that ask you some questions, and then tell you how many calories you will supposedly need. You can give them a try, but I have found the amount of calories that they told me to consume were too low for me to gain any weight.

A good way for me to discover how many calories I needed to gain weight was to multiply my body weight in pounds by 25. Since everyone is different, it is good to start out by multiplying by 20 first, then 22, and so on until you start gaining your 1 to 2 pounds a week. If you find that you are gaining 3 or more pounds per week, you might want to go back and subtract about 250 calories a day or so. You don't want to gain too much fat.

I will now let you in on another important thing that I had learned over the years. Eating more often will not really help you gain weight, and can actually promote weight loss. Eating small amounts of food more often will speed up your metabolism which in return, can actually make you lose weight. If you want to gain weight, chances are that you already have a fast metabolism. You don't want to raise it any higher.

I remember eating 500 calories 8 times a day until I noticed that I was actually losing weight. I decided to switch my plan to 1000 calories 4 times a day, and that is when my weight began to increase. Both of these diet plans include eating 4000 calories a day, but only one of them offered the result I was looking for. For this reason, I would not have more than 4 to five meals a day.

Eating larger portions fewer times a day might take some getting used to, but you can just start small and gradually build your way up. If you need 4000 calories a day, you can start out at 600 calories per meal, then on to 700, 800, and 900 until you reach 1000 calories in a single meal.

Many mass gaining programs out there will tell you to eat 6 to 8 times a day or more. This is a mistake that a lot of people make when they are trying to gain weight. They think that if they eat constantly, they will have no choice but to gain weight. After they fail to gain weight this way, they just give up.

The good news is that you don't have to spend all of your time eating all day, but you will need to get used to eating larger portions. Now you can be sure that you are eating enough calories without speeding up your metabolism.

Putting it Together

Now that you know about the types of nutrients that you should be eating, and how many calories you need to consume to gain weight the healthy way, it is time to give you an idea of exactly what a typical day should look like for you as far as your healthy weight gain diet goes.

For breakfast you might have 1 cup of oatmeal (measured uncooked), 3 eggs, 1 whole grain bagel with a couple tablespoons of olive oil, and a glass of juice. You can add cinnamon to the oatmeal for flavor. I also like to mix it with cream to make richer, and to add more calories.

This will give you at least 1000 calories, but as I stated earlier, if this amount of food feels overwhelming to you, just start with oatmeal and eggs, or just the bagel and eggs until you adjust.

At lunch you can have chicken and pasta. I like to use the smaller shell type of noodles, rather than long spaghetti noodles.

This way I can easily fit them inside a measuring cup to more accurately control how many calories I will get from them. I always liked to use boneless, skinless chicken that I would have grilled. I would be outside grilling all year long in rain, snow, sunshine, or darkness.

I even remember grilling when there was a lot of wind one day, trying not to let the flame go out. I was really motivated and persistent. You can substitute frozen precooked chicken for the grilled, skinless chicken, and just toss it in the oven, but it won't be as healthy. Next, you can add a tablespoon of olive oil to the pasta sauce for extra calories.

For dinner, I would have to say that steak has worked wonders for me. It didn't seem to matter if I had it with potatoes or corn on the cob for a side dish.

Because red meat seemed to be so good at promoting weight gain, I probably could have ate it with just about anything to see results. I understand that steak can be expensive to eat every day, but if you can afford to cut back in some other area financially, you will more easily gain weight this way.

If not, you can also have roast beef, meatloaf, or some other kind of meat. Just make sure to buy organic meat as often as you can in order to avoid the hormones.

A couple of peanut butter sandwiches and several glasses of whole milk can make an excellent before bedtime snack. The reason for this is because milk always seemed to last in my system longer.

The extra fat from the peanut butter would also make me feel full for a longer period of time than a simple bowl of cereal would.

This will ensure that you will be ready for the night long fast that you are about to undergo.

Some of these foods such as red meat, eggs, and whole milk might not be what your Doctor would recommend if you have a cholesterol problem. If that is the case, there are other options available.

One example is rice and beans. You can get plenty of carbohydrates from rice, while you can get a fair amount of protein by combining the rice and beans.

Once again, you can also add some olive oil to them for some extra calories. Use a large enough portion of rice, and you will have another high calorie meal. It is better to use brown rice when you can since it is healthier.

It is all about creativity and imagination.

You can switch things around, mix up food combinations to your own liking, and drop certain foods in favor of others.

The important thing is to make sure that your meals have a good balance of complex carbohydrates, the healthy kind of fat, and protein. You must also make sure that you are measuring your food in some way to make sure that you are getting enough calories.

Pizza is a good food to have on one of those days when you feel that you are unable to cook. It will help with your weight gain as it is high in carbohydrates, protein, and fat.

Remember to include enough organic fruits and vegetables with your diet as they contain fiber, vitamins, and minerals.

<u>What About Supplements?</u>

There is a wide variety of supplements to choose from out there that claim to give you results. I have tried many of supplements in the past with high hopes of them aiding in my weight gain quest.

The first one I tried was whey protein powder. After a few years, I realized that it was nothing special, and it is just basically meant to cover your protein requirements if you miss a meal. It did come in handy when I decided that the weight gainer supplements were not what I wanted as I mentioned in an earlier chapter.

I was able to make a better drink with the protein powder when I combined it with whole milk, olive oil, and honey. The sugar in the weight gainer drinks would get burned up fast, but the fat from the olive oil would burn slower, making it last longer. The small amount of honey I applied for flavor, contained very little sugar compared to the amount of sugar that was in the weight gainer supplements.

Putting things together in a blender is also a fast and convenient way to get extra calories.

I used to take vitamin supplements to help boost my immune system. I didn't notice any change in energy levels, or in how often I would get a cold or flu. It makes sense to just include organic fruits and vegetables in your diet to get the vitamins you need.

Other supplements I had tried included different types of amino acids, as well as other things that claimed to bring results. I spent plenty of money on these over the years until I realized that I never needed them. I am just glad that I have never tried steroids or anything like that.

Everyone is always looking for shortcuts in the form of a capsule or powder, when in fact, eating the right kinds of foods in large enough quantities can be like a shortcut in itself.

Whenever people talk about gaining weight, they usually like to base the conversation on supplements.

They always want to know about which supplements to take.

They should really focus on what kind of food to eat, how much food to eat, and how often to eat.

Lifting Weights to Gain Weight

By eating the right kinds of food in the right amounts, you will be able to put on some quality weight in a healthy way. But what if you want to put on some muscle mass as well? That is where working out with weights will come in.

There are so many different programs out there that can confuse you if you let them.

You might have stumbled across certain terminology such as drop sets, forced reps, negatives, and so on. These techniques are a more advanced form of exercise. Advanced techniques can still help, but they are best left for a later stage. When you are trying to add weight to your frame, it is better to stick with the basics.

Personally, I made the fastest progress by just sticking with straight sets, one after the other. I would gradually increase the weight on the exercises that I was doing, while making sure to give myself a few minutes of rest between sets.

As you increase the amount of weight that you are using on your exercises, you will have no choice but to gain more muscle mass.

It is important to understand that lifting weights without eating enough will not make you gain weight.

That is where I went wrong when I first started. Many people increase the weight over time on the exercises that they are doing because they think that it will give them more muscle mass which will then, amount to weight gain. Doing this will make you stronger and help give the muscles some more shape, but it won't help you to put on much weight.

The better thing to do is to make sure that you get your diet in order first by keeping track of your calories, making sure that you are eating enough without eating too often, so that you will not speed up your metabolism even more, and to make sure that you stay consistent enough to make something happen.

A lot of people keep lifting heavier and heavier weights without consuming enough calories to support what they are doing.

They gain some strength initially, but then they burn out. They think that maybe they just need a break. They take some time off from the gym, and then pick up where they left off.

But they still are unable to progress any further with the weight lifting because they are simply not taking in enough calories.

Once you put on some muscle mass by eating more calories and increasing the weights throughout the course of your workouts, you might notice your progress eventually come to a stop. This is where most people look to supplements for that extra edge, but you shouldn't have to do that.

Instead, you simply increase your calories even more. The extra weight that you gain from consuming more calories will allow you to deal with a heavier amount of weight. Calories are used for energy, and if you consume more of them than what you burn off, you will not only gain weight, but you will notice that you have more energy as well.

A large reason for the fatigue that I would feel at work was because I would not be hungry when it was really early in the morning. So I would just have a 90 calorie meal, and then I was out the door to face what was sometimes a 16 hour work day.

I know it is easier said than done, but if you can get up a little earlier to make a better breakfast, it will be worth it. It is still important to eat breakfast even when you are not hungry, just as it is important to drink water before running in a marathon, even if you do not yet feel thirsty at the time.

As with everything else, this can be done gradually. If you are used to just having a glass of juice for breakfast, try adding a slice of toast to that. Yogurt can be added the following week, and so on. Get yourself into the habit of eating a large enough breakfast to help you gain weight, and muscle mass.

So the idea is not to lift weights in hope of gaining weight through that alone. You will want to make sure that you are steadily gaining weight first through a high calorie diet, and then hit the weights to increase muscle size.

I am not suggesting that you gain a lot of fat, and then attempt to convert it into muscle. Fat cannot be translated into muscle. It is just better to make sure that you are headed in the right direction by gaining a few pounds through your diet first, and then proceeding with your weight lifting routine.

Which Exercises Are The Most Effective?

There are a couple of basic categories of exercises to choose from when it comes to working out.

These are known as compound, and isolation exercises.

Compound exercises work a group of muscles together. An example of a compound exercise would be the Bench Press. A Bench Press will primarily work the chest, but to a lesser degree, involve the triceps, and shoulders, as well.

Other compound exercises include Squats, and Pull-ups.

Isolation exercises, if done correctly, work one muscle group at a time. An example would be Dumbbell Kickbacks. This exercise will work your triceps without involving any other muscles.

It makes sense to stick with the compound movements when you are trying to gain weight, and put on muscle. You will be able to handle a heavier amount of weight when you do exercises that involve more than one muscle group.

Isolation exercises are used mostly for shaping a muscle, but not for building it up. If you insist on doing them, you should at least do them toward the end of your workout, since you will want to direct the majority of your energy towards the compound movements while you are fresh.

I was still able to gain muscle mass by incorporating some isolation exercises into my program, but I would not let them make up more than 25 percent of my routine.

Cardiovascular exercise can still be included in your weight gain program as well. Doing just 20 minutes every other day will not burn that many calories, but it will be good for heart health. Just make sure that you don't overdo it.

Now that you know about which types of movements you should be doing, it is time to get more specific about exactly what exercises should be used in a weight gain program.

Targeting Different Muscle Groups

Gaining weight will not work well if you just work on one muscle group, and then neglect the rest.

The Bench Press will work a large part of the upper body, but you must still remember to do exercises for the legs for balance. If all you do is squats, you will have an entire upper body that still looks skinny.

As you gain weight through food, the different body parts might start to fill out unevenly. You might notice that most of the weight is going to the legs, while your arms are still skinny.

Or maybe your arms are filling out, but your back is not as wide as you would like it to be. This is why it is good to do a full body workout. You can add an extra exercise to a certain muscle group that is falling behind.

Most people who are trying to gain weight, only do upper body exercises. Legs are half of the body, and if you don't include them in your weight gain routine, you could really hinder your progress.

So, to start with legs, Squats will work them really well. This is a big exercise that will allow you to lift more weight than most of the exercises you will do.

Squats primarily target the quadriceps. These can be followed by Leg Curls for the hamstrings. Calve Raises can close out the leg workout. You have now worked half of the body just by doing a few exercises.

The Bench Press will be the most effective exercise to build mass for the chest. This is another exercise that will allow you to use heavier weight than most other exercises. It is important not to arch your back during this exercise. Keep your back flat against the bench, and use the chest to drive up the weight.

Pull-ups have always been my go to exercise for the back. It can be challenging at first to make sure that your arms are not doing all the work.

You need to feel your back working during this exercise in order for it to be effective. Just tense up the muscles in your back while you are performing this exercise until you feel them working throughout the motion. Pullovers can follow the Pull-ups in order to hit the back from a different angle.

The Pullover machines at the gym have worked very well for me, but these can also be done at home by lying on the floor using a barbell. I do not do Barbell Rows because I believe that they can be bad for the back in the long run.

Over-the-head pressing movements can be used along with lateral raises for the shoulders. It's usually better to stick with dumbbells when it comes to shoulder exercises. I don't like to lift barbells over my head due to the lack of range of motion, but this is a personal choice.

Biceps and triceps will usually grow from the chest and back exercises that you are doing. Bench presses will involve the triceps secondarily, while pull-ups will end up using the biceps as well as back.

Even if you do a good job at isolating the back muscles during pull-ups, the biceps will still be involved to some degree.

But if you want to give these muscles some extra work, you can do Standing Barbell Curls for biceps and Close-Grip Bench Presses for triceps.

Customizing Your Workout Program

Even after doing a full body workout, you may still find that certain muscle groups are responding while others are not where you would like them to be.

If you are lacking in upper chest development, you could benefit by adding incline bench presses to your routine.

Or maybe your upper arms have gained size, but now your forearms are out of balance in relation to them. You can add Barbell Reverse Curls and Behind-The-Back Wrist Curls to help correct that problem.

Whatever the case may be, you will simply have to make adjustments to correct the problem that you are experiencing. You can add another exercise to a muscle group that is not responding, or you can start doing extra sets to give it more work.

It is a good idea not to do more than 12 sets each for triceps, biceps, shoulders, and forearms. These muscle groups are smaller, and therefore, don't require as much work.

Chest, back, and legs can be worked by doing 15 sets for each. However you want to do it is up to you and your individual needs. Just try to stay within that set frame. You might do 8 sets of squats, and then 7 sets of leg curls; or 5 sets of squats, 5 sets of leg curls, and 5 sets of the leg press. If your quadriceps need more work, do more squats. If your hamstrings need more work, do more leg curls.

The amount of repetitions you do for each set should be within the 8 to 12 range. Start out with an amount of weight that you can only do 8 reps with. Then, rest for a couple minutes before doing 8 reps again.

Just continue that cycle until you finish all your sets. The next workout, you can go for 10 reps for each set. You add about 5 pounds to the exercise once you are able to do 12 reps for each set with only slight difficulty. If it still feels rather difficult to complete the 12 reps, it is not time to add weight yet.

You might do better training chest and back together, or training back and biceps in the same workout.

Keep in mind that biceps are involved in many back exercises, so you might overwork them if you do them in the same workout as your back. You might have to try both before you decide which you like better.

Generally, each muscle group should be worked once or twice a week. Any more than that, you are mostly just wasting your time, since you will need time to recover.

Working out more often will keep the muscles looking hard, but it won't do much to help you gain extra weight. Any muscle group that is falling behind can be worked twice a week while the rest can be worked once a week.

HOW TO BUILD MUSCLE FAST
GET THE RESULTS YOU WANT WITHOUT TAKING SUPPLEMENTS

By DAVID A. HUNTER

Disclaimer:

The views expressed within this book are those of the author alone. The information contained within this book is based on the opinions, experiences, and observations of the author and is provided "AS-IS".

No warranties of any kind are made. Neither the author nor publisher are engaged in rendering professional services of any kind. The information contained within this book is not intended to treat, cure, or prevent any kind of health, medical, or any other condition. The information contained within this book should not be used to replace the advice of a competent professional. You should always speak with your doctor before beginning any kind of diet or exercise program. Neither the author nor publisher will assume liability or responsibility for any loss or damage related directly or indirectly to the information contained within this book.

The author has attempted to be as accurate as possible with the information contained within this book. Neither the author nor publisher will assume responsibility or liability for any errors, omissions, inconsistencies, or inaccuracies.

Why Should You Even Care About Building Muscle?

There are many people that claim to not see the benefits of building muscle.

Now that there are machines to do the heavy lifting for us, some people are unable to understand why anyone would want to build muscle.

The bottom line is that there are benefits to building muscle.

Personally, I have experienced these benefits in my life, and so can you.

We also use our muscles all the time.

We use our muscles when we are lifting, climbing, pushing things, pulling things, carrying things, or doing any type of manual labor. Since we are constantly using our muscles, it makes sense to build them up to their fullest potential.

Many people seem to be more concerned about their financial health and less concerned about their physical health.

Building muscle can provide you with a strong foundation. You just need to know the right way to do it in order to see results.

You will carry the same body with you throughout your entire life, so why not make the best of it?

Packing on some quality muscle to your frame is a great way to make the best of it.

You also probably want to build muscle fast in order to reap the benefits as soon as you can.

Although you won't reap all the benefits overnight, you can build some quality muscle pretty fast with the right diet and exercise program.

There are short-term and long-term benefits to building muscle.

It could be years before you notice the long-term benefits, but I remember noticing short-term benefits after my very first workout.

Here are some examples of short-term benefits that you might notice right away:

-Feeling stronger than you did the day before, even though you might not actually be stronger yet

-Feeling better about yourself for having the discipline to workout

-Feeling like you have accomplished something important

-Experiencing a release of tension

-Feeling less angry, less irritable, less depressed, less anxious, or less sad

-Feeling like the muscles have gotten harder, even though they haven't actually grown bigger yet

The long-term benefits are even better. The length of time it takes to achieve the long-term benefits will depend on how consistent you are

Here are some examples of long-term benefits that you might notice:

-Increased strength

-Increased muscle mass

-Increased muscle definition

-Higher self-esteem

-More confidence

-Better health

While I do believe that muscle building is a popular magnet for narcissists, I know for a fact that not everyone that does it is a narcissist.

Some of the best things in life will always attract a lot of narcissists. There are also plenty of evil people who have a lot of money, but that doesn't make money bad. Having a lot of money does not make you evil, and having a good body does not make you a narcissist.

You can't deny the benefits that come along with muscle building, just like you can't deny the benefits of having more money.

Building muscle has helped me tremendously over the years. If you practice using good form on the exercises, not only will you build muscle, you will become less vulnerable to injuries as well. I used to get lower back pain a lot, but it finally went away after I started doing DEADLIFTS, which seemed to help strengthen that area.

It's a good feeling to be solid and full of strength.

As long as you don't overdo it, muscle building can make your daily tasks seem a lot easier. Grocery bags feel lighter, your posture improves, and you feel ready to take on the world.

Turning your body into a powerhouse can make you feel much more energetic and full of life. Many of the coolest and most laid back people I have ever known, all happened to be strong and muscular. Believe me. It's not just a coincidence.

It enhances everything and makes your life better. It's like putting on a special pair of glasses that allows you to see even better than the standard 20/20 vision. Your outlook on life can drastically improve.

The thing about money is that you never really see it that much. You either spend it, keep it in your wallet, or put it into you bank account.

Once you spend the money, it's gone, and then you have to work to get it back. The good thing about having a good body is that you get to carry it with you all the time. It's always there, and as long as you stay consistent with your diet and exercise program, you can continue to reap the benefits 24/7.

That's why I feel that health is even more important than financial abundance.

Don't go broke over trying to build muscle, but make sure that you are treating your health with the same level of priority as the other important things in your life.

If people would start taking their health as seriously as they took their finances, they would get results a lot faster.

Planning Everything Out And Writing It All Down

When you are starting out, it really helps to keep a record of what you are doing and what you are trying to accomplish.

This will become less important as you get closer to where you want to be with your goals, but it's highly recommended in the early stages of your journey.

Don't make the same mistake I did by trying to guess at how many calories you are consuming or trying to remember how much weight you lifted the week before.

When it comes to your diet, keep track of how many calories you are taking in, and how much protein, carbohydrates, and fat you are consuming. Nutrition is a big part of muscle building, so don't neglect keeping track of it.

When it comes to your workout program, write down all of the exercises you are doing, and keep track of the amount of weight you are lifting, as well as the number of sets and reps you are doing. It can be difficult to remember the exact amount of weight you were using for all of your different exercises.

There won't be much of a point in working out with 5lbs less than what you were lifting during your last workout session.

Don't waste your time in the gym just because you didn't keep track of what you were doing the last time. You also don't want to risk an injury by accidentally loading more weight on the barbell than what you are ready for.

Not keeping track of my measurements was another mistake I made when I first got into muscle building. I used to just check my body weight on the scale without measuring my waist, arms, etc.

The idea is to gain as much muscle as possible without adding too much fat to your frame. But you won't know how much fat you are gaining if you don't even measure your waist.

You can also purchase a caliper to get a better idea of where your body fat levels are.

Although, it's not necessary, writing things down shows that you are serious. When you write something down, it sends a signal to your brain that you are getting ready for something important.

Personally, I had good results when I was keeping track of everything and writing it all down. You don't have to obsess over writing absolutely everything down all the time, but writing down what you can will definitely help you more than you might think.

<u>Make Sure Your Mind Is Where It Needs To Be</u>

If you only remember one chapter from this book, make it this one. If you want the physical aspect of yourself to change for the better, you have to change your thinking for the better.

It didn't matter what other people told me. They might think that you don't have what it takes to build muscle.

Whether it's done intentionally or unintentionally, certain people might not be supportive of what you are doing. But as long as your mind is in the right place, you can bypass all of the negativity that you might happen to encounter.

People would tell me that I would actually "burn muscle" if I worked out for longer than an hour a day.

When I told them about my plans, they would say, "Good luck with that." It won't matter what they say when your desire and persistence is strong enough. I knew what appealed to me, and I knew what didn't appeal to me.

It all starts with having the motivation to improve yourself. You will still have to take action, but it will be much easier to take action when your mind is in the right place.

Don't turn health and fitness into an obsession, but make sure you stay consistent in your efforts. Consistency will often follow an excitement to achieve your goals.

Between workouts, you should be looking forward to the next one. When you feel like skipping a meal, you need to remember that building muscle will require you to eat regularly. Keep a picture in your mind of what you would like to look like.

If you can stay consistently motivated, your thoughts can lead you to the necessary actions to achieve your muscle building goals.

The things you choose to keep on your mind can make or break you and your progress.

There are still plenty of things to go over when you are trying to build muscle. You will still need to do the right things aside from putting your mind in the right place, but believing in yourself will help you break through barriers that get in the way.

The Best Muscle Building Exercises For Fast Results

Although different individuals believe in different exercises, I am going to go over the ones that seemed to have worked the best for myself, as well as other people I have known.

I have had my share of experience with different exercises over the years.

Eventually, I was able to separate the good ones from the mediocre ones. I have also worked out with a lot of people, and as a result, I have seen which muscle building exercises most people seem to respond to the most.

Some of the exercises are common, and some of the exercises are not so commonly practiced in gyms these days.

But keep in mind that many of the effective exercises are usually the same ones that are the most challenging. Taking the easy route is not the answer in this case.

Here are the exercises that I have found to work best for building muscle fast:

-Squats
-Lying leg curls
-Chin Ups
-DEADLIFTS
-Bench Press
-Incline Bench Press
-DUMBBELL FLYS
-Shoulder Presses
-Lateral Raises
-TRICEPS CABLE PUSHDOWNS
-Close-Grip Bench Press
-Lying Triceps Extensions
-Standing Barbell Curls
-Incline Dumbbell Curls
-Reverse Barbell Curls
-Behind-The-Back Wrist Curls
-Standing Calf Raises

These fourteen exercises should serve you well when you are trying to pack on as much muscle as you can in the shortest amount of time possible.

These exercises are especially good for beginners, but unless you plan on becoming a professional bodybuilder, I don't see why you should ever really need to add any other exercises to your routine, even as you become more advanced. If the exercises work, why change them?

If you do insist on trying some other exercises just to prevent boredom and keep things interesting, there are also some exercises that are worth doing.

Here are some additional exercises that I have found to not be quite as effective for fast muscle building, but can still be beneficial:

-Lunges
-Front Squats
-Seated Calf Raises
-Pullovers
-LAT MACHINE PULLDOWNS

-Dips
-Seated Triceps Presses
-Alternate Dumbbell Curls

These exercises can give you an extra boost in your muscle development without slowing you down. They can improve your results, but you shouldn't give them priority over the other exercises.

I would avoid any exercise that has you holding onto only one light dumbbell at a time. Some examples of those exercises are:

-Dumbbell Kickbacks
-Dumbbell Pullovers
-Concentration Curls
-One-Arm Triceps Extensions

These exercises will not allow you to use much weight. Increased muscle size will come from lifting the heavy weights, not the light ones.

However, if you are able to use a fair amount of weight on these exercises without sacrificing good form, it shouldn't be a problem.

A popular exercise for building muscle that I left out was Bent-Over Rows. This exercise can work your back really well, but over a period of time, I believe it ends up doing more harm than good. Bending over like that already leaves you in a vulnerable position.

Combine that vulnerable position with holding on to a heavy barbell or set of dumbbells, and you are making an enemy out of your back.

A much more powerful and beneficial exercise is the DEADLIFT. It works the hamstrings to a large degree, but it can also thicken the lower back. It also allows you to use heavier weight.

It might not work the same exact area of the back, but it will help you to build more muscle overall. Real strength is developed through the core exercises. It is well known that it's better to lift with your legs, not with your back. The DEADLIFT will allow you to lift with your hamstrings while working certain parts of the back.

If you insist on doing rows, try to find a gym that offers a machine that you can do them on. Machine rows and seated cable rows will allow you to keep your back in a better position.

I also haven't mentioned any abdominal exercises. This is because I believe that the best thing you can do to develop the abdominal muscles is to reduce your body fat.

I also believe that the majority of your body fat reduction will come from the right diet, not necessarily the right exercise. Get your diet in order first, and then pick whichever abdominal exercise you like best.

Practice Good Form In Order To Form Good Muscles

Before you can build muscle in a safe way while minimizing the chance of getting injured, you will need to make sure that you are using the right form.

I know how easy it is to get excited about building muscle, and just wanting to jump into the exercises without carefully considering how to do them the right way.

But you will be much better off taking the time to slowly go through the motions of the exercises with very light weight or even no weight at all before you begin your actual workout program.

Master the general movement of the exercises before you start adding any weight to them.

When I first started out, I was doing very high reps with light weight. I was able to develop excellent form on my exercises because I stayed patient and started off slow. Start out as light as you need to, and don't increase the weight until you get the hang of it.

Here are some tips to follow:

-When you are Bench Pressing, don't arch your back in any way. To prevent your back from leaving the bench, try to keep your legs flat, instead of bent.

-When you are doing any kind of biceps curls, keep your elbows slightly bent when you reach the bottom part of the movement. Don't allow your arms to extend themselves down all the way. Stretching them out at the bottom part of the movement will increase your chance of getting injured. When you get to the top of the movement, squeeze the biceps and hold that position for a second before lowering the weight back down. Keep your back straight and don't swing the weight around. You can practice doing curls by keeping your back up against a wall in order to keep it from moving during the exercise.

-When you do squats, don't go too heavy. The excessive amount of weight can be bad for the knees. The Squat is known as a power exercise, but you shouldn't have to go lower than 6 reps. As long as you do the exercise the right way with really good form, you can still get the results you are looking for.

-You should try to use dumbbells for your shoulder presses. The barbell can force your shoulders into an unusual position that can leave you feeling really tight and restricted. Dumbbells can make you feel a bit more loose when you are doing shoulder presses. You also won't have to worry about slamming the barbell into your head.

-Squeeze the back muscles when you are doing back exercises. When I first started working out, it took me a while to actually feel my back doing the work on the back exercises. My biceps would take over while my back would hardly get worked at all. Since you need to use your arms to do the back exercises, it can be difficult to make sure that they aren't doing all the work. This problem can be solved if you simply focus on the back muscles that you are trying to work. Start squeezing the back muscles as if you were trying to flex them, and maintain constant tension on them throughout each set.

-It's a good idea to not use a lot of weight on the triceps exercises. Triceps exercises can place a lot of tension on the elbows. I had a friend that used to like going really heavy on triceps exercises, but when he did a bigger exercise, such as the Bench Press, he would go light. It's important that you don't mix up the isolation exercises with the compound movements. The Bench Press will work the chest, triceps, and shoulders. Since you have different muscle groups involved in the Bench Press, it makes since to go a bit heavier. But going heavy on an isolation exercise such as TRICEPS PUSHDOWNS will only cause the wrong muscles to do the work. Isolation exercises are not intended to involve more than one muscle group at a time. Go heavier on the compound movements, and go lighter on the isolation exercises.

    -Don't do exercises or stretches that require you to bend too far at the waist. Don't do Bent-Over Rows, Hamstring Stretches where you reach down and touch the ground, etc.

    -Remember to lift with your knees when you are picking up weights off the ground.

    Building your foundation is essential when you want to add muscle mass onto your frame. Mastering the correct lifting techniques will help you to build that foundation. Failing to use the correct form for the exercises is like trying to build a house with the wrong tools. Using good form and the right amount of weight on the exercises will ensure that your workouts are safer and more productive.

How Often Should You Workout When You Want To Build Muscle Fast?

Over-training is a concern that many bodybuilders have. But I don't believe that everyone has the same recuperation abilities.

What might seem like *over*-training to some might seem like *under*-training to others and vice versa.

I have experimented with many different workout programs over the years. I have worked some muscle groups everyday, while I have worked other muscle groups just once a week.

Excessive soreness, muscle spasms, lack of gains, and lack of motivation to work out are some of the signs that you have over-trained.

It will take some time and experience to determine what workout routine is best for you, but there are some general "rules" to consider.

If your main goal is to just gain weight and bulk up, you will need to keep in mind that excessive physical activity will burn an excessive amount of calories. Gaining weight has a lot more to do with nutrition than it has to do with exercise. It's usually unnecessary to work each muscle group more than once a week when your main goal is to gain weight.

When you want to gain muscle mass fast and look more defined, it makes sense to work the muscles often enough to build them up in as short of a time as possible, but not often enough to strain them.

Building muscle mass can be more complex than simply gaining weight, especially when you are trying to do it fast.

If you worked at a job for 18 hours straight, you would be exhausted by the end of the day. You would probably stop being productive after the 6th hour or so. The next 12 hours would, for the most part, be a waste of time. But if you worked for 6 hours, took the next 12 hours off, and then came back for another 6 hours of work, that would change everything. In the same 24 hour period, you could get 12 hours of productive work done, instead of getting 6 hours of productive work done. Taking more time off would actually allow you to get more work done.

Even when you are trying to do something fast, it's important not to rush things along. I you want to gain as much muscle as you can in the shortest time possible, it makes sense to lift weights often, but for fairly short periods of time.

The frequency of your workout sessions will depend on how sore you usually get, and the length of time it takes you to recover.

You want to work the muscle again as soon as it recovers. Why waste time? If the muscles have already recovered from your previous workout, that means they are just sitting there waiting for you to break them down again.

Think of it as an open window of opportunity.

There is a time and place for everything. You will have time to rest when you are sore. After you have recovered, it's time to work out again.

I have noticed that working each muscle group once a week would make me feel like I lost my momentum. I would get sore more often, and I just wasn't making any progress that way. The reps wouldn't increase.

Working each muscle group three times a week or more helped me make faster progress, but it took up a lot of my time. Working each muscle group at least 3 times a week also forced me to combine a lot of muscle groups into one workout session. This can be very demanding.

I began to switch my workout routine to something that was more accommodating. I decided to work each muscle group twice a week. I was making the same amount of progress as I was making when I would work each muscle group 3 times a week or more. The difference was that it no longer took up as much of my time as it used to.

Working each muscle group twice a week will ensure that you are building muscle as fast as you can without wasting your time. This will allow yourself enough time for recovery without having to sacrifice your momentum.

Again, you will have to monitor your progress regularly. Perhaps working each muscle group once a week will be sufficient.

The Amount Of Reps You Should Be Doing To Build Muscle Fast

When I first started working out, I would do very high reps. I would do 1 set of about 60 reps, and then my workout would be over. I didn't gain any muscle this way, but it did help me to develop good form.

I decided to increase the weight to the point where I would not be able to do much more than 10 reps. I was still keeping the sets really low, but now I was only doing about 10 reps at a time. I was finally starting to see some progress, but only a little bit. I started adding more exercises to my workout routine, but this didn't help much. I was still not seeing the results that I was looking for.

After some more experimentation, I realized that the amount of sets you do are just as important as the amount of reps you do.

As a beginner, I would do just a few sets per exercise. I was also doing only a couple of exercises per muscle group. For the most part, I was doing 4 to 6 sets total per muscle group. I didn't have to worry about overdoing it when I worked out this way, but I didn't have much to show for all of my hard work either. I had experimented with different rep ranges, but I didn't start making any major progress until I started adding more sets to my routine.

Doing high reps with low sets did not bring me any gains, and doing low sets with low reps did not help much.

Doing high sets and medium reps worked best for packing on muscle fast. Doing sets with high reps seemed to be a waste of time, while doing low sets just didn't seem to be enough. Try to keep your reps around 8 to15 per set, and your sets around 4 to 15 per muscle group.

You might wish to lower your sets for the smaller muscle groups, and you might wish to do some more sets for the big muscle groups.

Don't forget to include at least one warm-up set. A typical warm-up set should include about 12 to 20 reps.

What Should Your Workout Routine Look Like For Fast Results?

Using the recommended exercises that are listed in an earlier chapter, your workout routine might look something like this:

Monday, Thursday- Legs, Calves

Squats- 5 sets of 6-15 reps
Leg Curls- 5 sets of 10 reps
Lunges- 3 sets of 8-10 reps
Standing Calf Raises- 4 sets of 6-15 reps

Tuesday, Friday- Arms, Shoulders

Standing Barbell Curls- 4 sets of 6-10 reps
Incline Dumbbell Curls- 4 sets of 8 reps
TRICEPS CABLE PUSHDOWNS- 4 sets of 12-20 reps
Close-Grip Bench Press- 4 sets of 8-15 reps
Reverse Barbell Curls- 4 sets of 8 reps
Behind-The-Back Wrist Curls- 4 sets of 10 reps
Shoulder Presses- 4 sets of 8 reps
Lateral Raises- 4 sets of 8 reps

Wednesday, Saturday- Chest, Back, and Abdominal

Bench Press- 5 sets of 4-10 reps
Incline Bench Press- 5 sets of 8 reps
Chin Ups (Wide-grip)- 4 sets of 10-12 reps
Chin Ups (Close-grip)- 4 sets of 10 reps
Pullovers- 3 sets of 12 reps
DEADLIFTS- 2 sets of 4-12 reps

The abdominal exercise can be whichever you prefer, but remember, the abdominal muscles will only be visible if you have a low amount of body fat in that area.

Don't bother trying to overdo it with the abdominal exercises in hopes of having better muscle development. Pick one exercise, and do about 4 sets of 20 to 25 reps.

The bigger exercises are usually more effective when you do them with lower reps. That is why your reps can be a little bit lower with an exercise such as the Bench Press or DEADLIFT.

Remember to start out with very light weight on all of the exercises, and then gradually increase the amount of weight on them over time to allow yourself to adjust. Even if you feel like you are strong enough to lift heavier, your joints might not be ready. It's best to be patient if you want to minimize the chance of an injury.

If six days a week is too much for you, try doing the chest, back, and abdominal workout just once a week, legs and calves once a week, and the arms and shoulders workout once a week.

Nutrition is more important than the actual workout routine, anyway.

If you are still sore from a previous workout, take as much time off as you need.

<u>**How To Separate Hype From What Is Real**</u>

Even with experience, it can be confusing when you are trying to figure out what really works and what doesn't.

When I was in my teens, I went into a store that sold supplements. The Salesman/Owner was trying to convince me to buy a product that was supposed to increase your "pump." He never even mentioned anything about building muscle or gaining weight. I guess the pump was supposed to lead to muscle gains or something like that.

I tried my share of different supplements, but none of them really worked. The only supplements that seemed to do anything were the ones with caffeine in them. These products would have all kinds of "special" vitamins and amino acids in them, but the only thing I really noticed was the caffeine. They would give me extra energy for my workouts, but I could have saved money if I just had coffee instead.

CREATINE is another product that became popular, but I still can't understand why. You basically gain 5 lbs of water weight when you cycle onto it, and then you lose the 5lbs after you cycle off. You also have to drink a lot of water when you are on it. I can also experienced bad side effects from the "loading phase."

Even when you get a pump, that doesn't mean you are automatically getting bigger and stronger. Getting bigger will require you to consume more calories than what you burn off, and getting stronger will require you to lift heavier weights with the correct form.

I remember doing a bunch of consecutive sets without stopping for rest. I would do the Standing Barbell Curl, Reverse Curls, Standing Alternate Dumbbell Curls, and then Concentration Curls without resting in between the exercises. I would see what a huge pump I was getting, so I kept doing it. After months went by and I still hadn't really gotten any bigger or stronger, I decided to ditch that idea of doing so many nonstop sets. I realized that getting a really good pump will not necessarily lead you to bigger and better things.

It's more effective to just eat more, rest between sets, and gradually add weight to the exercises over time. Don't make it a priority to get a pump. Make it a priority to gain some strength and build muscle. Don't just pump up the muscles, build, strengthen, and develop them.

You will usually need to increase your overall body weight if you want to gain muscle. I used to eat a lot of protein, while carefully monitoring my carbohydrate and fat intake. I was hoping to gain pure muscle by emphasizing protein and minimizing carbohydrates and fats. I also took supplements that were supposed to help me put on muscle. I did gain some muscle weight, but it was only 5 lbs after a whole year.

If you want to gain muscle fast, you will have to be willing to gain some fat as well. You can try to gain pure muscle if you want, but you will most likely lose your patience and become disappointed with the results.

Many people want to gain muscle and lose fat at the same time, but this is not very realistic. It would be like pulling yourself in two different directions. You would go nowhere fast. It is much better to stay focused on one thing at a time. If you want to lose fat and build muscle, it is best to try to gain the muscle first, and then trim down on the fat later. So if you weigh 160 lbs, you might bulk up to 180lbs, and then trim down to 170lbs. You would be 10 lbs heavier than when you first started, but this time, you wouldn't be carrying around so much weight in terms of fat. It would be more difficult and time consuming however, to try to go straight up to 170lbs without putting on any fat.

If you want to get bigger, spend your money on food, not supplements. If you want to get stronger, spend your time studying the correct lifting techniques, not on studying the newest supplement information.

Bad Days Can Actually Be Good Days In Disguise

There will be many days when you just won't feel like working out. You might find it easy enough to get yourself motivated once or twice a week, but it can be challenging to maintain this motivation each day, week after week.

There would be times when I would feel like skipping a workout. Fortunately, the less motivated I would feel, the harder I would try to get myself into a good mood. It's similar to perspiration. If you feel comfortable temperature-wise, the body just sits back and does nothing. But if you subject yourself to a lot of heat, the body will respond by causing you to sweat to help cool you off.

Sometimes we need to experience a bad day in order to help us remember the things that are really important to us. Sometimes we lose sight of why we are doing what we are doing, and we just end up going through the motions without any passion or enthusiasm.

It's alright to take some time off from working out if you need to. You can take several weeks off if you need to, but make sure that you plan it that way. Don't procrastinate by saying that you are going to do something, and then not doing it. When you plan to workout, stick to it. When you plan on taking time off, stick to that. Unless you get sick, injured, or you have to deal with an emergency, don't cancel a workout that you had planned on.

If you ever played sports, you know that you have to try harder when you are going up against a really tough team. Our true capabilities are not tested when we play the easier teams. Even if we don't win, we usually end up doing a lot better than we thought we would.

You might miss a really awesome, productive workout if you allow negative thoughts to push you around. Don't allow a lack of motivation to get the best of you. Most people like to wait for their motivation to return before they take action, but sometimes you have to take action in order to bring back your motivation.

It's What You Do Outside The Gym That Counts

Obviously, working out will play a big role when you are building muscle. You will need to break down the muscles through exercise before they can grow back bigger. It's also important that you do the right exercises at the right frequency.

But there is another side to the muscle building equation, and if you don't master it, you will never make the kind of progress that you are looking for.

Outside the gym, you will need to make sure that you are:

-Consuming enough calories to support what you are doing

-Drinking enough water to stay hydrated

-Getting at least 7 hours of sleep each night

-Giving yourself enough time to unwind

In order to gain muscle fast, you will need to gain some weight. In order to gain weight, you will need to increase the amount of calories you are consuming. Stick to foods that are filling, and you should do fine.

You must remember to drink water outside of the gym, not just when you're at the gym. I have had good results from drinking 50-80 ounces of water a day, but that is just the average. You will need more water, if you lose more of it, so make sure that you take notice of hot weather, manual labor, etc, and make adjustments accordingly.

It's always good to give yourself some time to unwind at least once a day. The body has a difficult time trying to carry out the things it needs to do (including repairing muscle tissue) when you are always putting it under some kind of stress.

Sitting outside or watching something funny can help more than you might think.

I have always liked to say, "Rest is good, sleep is better." Rest and relaxation are good, but they won't be enough if you aren't getting at least 7 hours of sleep per night.

Some people can get away with only sleeping 5 hours a night all year long, but not everyone has that luxury. Sometimes you might still feel tired, regardless of how much or how little sleep you got the night before. If you are unsure of how much sleep you really need, try to aim for about 7-8 hours a night.

Building muscle is not as easy as building a house. When you build a house, you can stop working on it at the end of the day, forget about it overnight, and then pick up the next day where you left off. Building muscle requires constant attention.

The work never really stops.

When you're not working out, you are either eating, drinking water, sleeping, or thinking about your next workout to keep yourself motivated and focused. You shouldn't be obsessing about anything, but you must always keep your goals in the front of your mind where you can see them.

Feel free to change things around until you find something that suits you. Although many people of different shapes and sizes have benefited from the principles within this book, it's not good to feel confined to any particular thing. Switch things around until you find something that fits.

Even if you aren't gaining muscle as fast as you would like, instead of getting frustrated, stay focused. Frustration will just make things worse.

Keep practicing persistence, and wait for it to happen.

HOW TO BURN FAT
BEST WAYS TO BURN FAT WITHOUT USING SUPPLEMENTS

By DAVID A. HUNTER

Disclaimer:

The views expressed within this book are those of the author alone. The information contained within this book is based on the opinions, experiences, and observations of the author and is provided "AS-IS". No warranties of any kind are made. Neither the author nor publisher are engaged in rendering professional services of any kind. This book is not intended to treat, cure, or prevent any kind of health, medical, or any other condition. The information contained within this book should not be used to replace the advice of a competent professional. You should always speak with your Doctor before you begin any kind of diet or exercise program. Neither the author nor publisher will assume liability or responsibility for any loss or damage related directly or indirectly to the information contained within this book.

The author has attempted to be as accurate as possible with the information contained within this book. Neither the author nor publisher will assume liability or responsibility for any errors, omissions, inconsistencies, or inaccuracies.

<u>Managing Your Expectations When You Want To Burn Fat</u>

There are so many people out there that are interested in burning fat. Many people fail, but only a small percentage of people succeed.

Burning fat can be challenging enough as it is, but keeping it off is an even greater challenge.

It requires hard work, while maintaining your ideal body weight requires discipline. But hard work and discipline do not have to be as horrible as you might imagine them to be.

It's similar to taking a trip across the country. If you had to drive 2,000 miles just to do a ton of work for free, you would probably see the 2,000 mile journey as a chore. But if you were traveling 2,000 miles to go on the best vacation of your life, you wouldn't have much of a problem with traveling so far.

Both of these scenarios involve traveling the same distance, but only one destination is a favorable one.

If burning fat is something that you really want to do, it shouldn't have to feel like a chore. Just like an artist's passion shouldn't have to feel like work, a burning desire should not feel painful to attain. Burning fat is the objective, but making sure that you don't gain it back is more like a lifestyle.

If you want health and fitness to be a part of your lifestyle, you will need to view health and fitness in a positive light. I want this book to help you realize that your journey does not have to be a horrible one.

The idea is to make your healthy lifestyle fun so that you will be able to continue it throughout the course of your life.

Quitting is not necessarily the result of hard work, but the result of an inability to fully appreciate what you are doing.

We need to be more understanding with ourselves and our goals. Oftentimes, we set our expectations too high, and then we feel like we "failed" when we don't achieve our goals.

We feel like we failed when we really just had the wrong expectations.

Before you can manage your expectations, you will need to take a look at your options. You can lose weight fast, but then you will be more likely to just gain it all back. You can severely restrict your food intake, but then you will be hungry all the time.

There has to be balance in your life. If you want long term results, you need to find something that is effective, yet comfortable enough to suit your needs. You will need to be positive, yet realistic about your goals.

Don't settle for less than what you're worth, but don't set yourself up for disappointment.

Ideally, you should try to burn fat without losing muscle mass in the process. The quickest route to burning fat is not always the best one.

I remember losing about 10 lbs in a month, but I also noticed that my strength had decreased as well. I found myself lifting about 20 lbs less than I normally would on most of my exercises. After going back to reevaluate what I did, I started over again. I gained the weight back, and then burned off the fat without losing any strength while I was doing it.

One of the tricks is to not try to rush things along before they are ready to happen. I know that you want to get everything done right now, but you need to think about long term results. Be patient now, and then be happy with the results later.

Personally, I have never really experienced many benefits with supplements.

Caffeine can decrease your appetite and allow you to work out harder, but it is also addictive. It can also cause irritability, nervousness, and sleep problems. Most people like to buy supplements because they are always looking for fast and easy results. I used to be one of these people. When I finally decided to ditch them for good, my results proved that I never really needed them in the first place.

Instead of buying a ton of supplements, you would be better off spending your money on healthy food.

If you manage your expectations correctly, you will realize that you don't need supplements because there is no such thing as fast and easy results when it comes to burning fat.

This book will go over some of the best ways I have found to burn fat. The more of these ideas you apply, the better your results will be.

Aiming For Long-Term Results To Maximize Your Benefits

After getting your expectations in order, you should now understand the importance of aiming for long-term results. Short-term results are similar to empty promises. They give you a small boost at first, but then they let you down later.

Burning fat should not have to take you the rest of your life, but eliminating the constant desire to have everything right now can save you a lot of frustration.

In my experience, losing more than a couple of lbs a week would always backfire. I was only able to accomplish this by eating about 40% of what I would usually eat.

By cutting down on my food intake in such a drastic way, I would start to feel lightheaded, and of course, extremely hungry.

It was very frustrating trying to burn fat this way. I would not only have less energy, but I would get a much stronger urge to eat unhealthy food as well. It's almost as if I was trying to make up for lost time by eating more unhealthy food than ever.

When you are trying to burn fat, losing 1-2 lbs a week is plenty. Losing 4-8 lbs a month will ensure that you are making progress without doing anything unhealthy or counterproductive.

Remember, the trick is to like what you're doing. Losing more than a couple of lbs a week will most likely require you to do a lot of things that you don't want to do. You should aim for long-term results by losing weight gradually, not drastically.

I know that it's easier said than done, but patience is a must. If you are losing 1 lb a week, you are already seeing results, so there is no reason to try rushing your way through everything. Just remember that 1 lb a week can add up to 8 lbs in a couple of months.

Keep in mind that working out with weights can cause you to gain weight due to the extra muscle tissue.

This is where measuring your waist comes in handy. If the numbers on the scale stay the same or increase, while your waist size decreases, you can rest assured that you are burning fat. You might also wish to purchase a caliper.

There is usually an instruction packet included with the caliper that tells you what to do, so all you have to do is follow it. Since there are other factors to consider when you are trying to burn fat, you shouldn't let the numbers on the scale bother you too much.

It can be difficult to stay motivated every single day. Sticking with a certain diet 7 days a week can be very challenging. For this reason, you should allow yourself 1 or 2 days a week to consume food that isn't part of your fat-burning diet plan.

That doesn't mean you should eat extremely unhealthy food for 2 days straight, but most people are much more likely to get better results when they allow themselves to take breaks.

Having pizza once a week can make things easier on you in the long term. In a way, you are almost restoring yourself by taking a break from your usual diet.

Regardless of what you are doing, it's always important to give yourself enough breaks. Without adequate breaks, productivity can suffer. That includes allowing yourself to enjoy life when you are trying to burn fat.

One of the best ways to burn fat is to make sure that you don't burn yourself out. Think of it as a marathon, not a sprint.

If you are too hard on yourself now, what will you do later when you are all out of energy? It's basically like taking one step back now to avoid falling three steps back later. Just like you need to take breaks at work in order to stay productive, you need to take breaks from your goals in order to achieve them.

Instead of feeling guilty about "cheating on your diet", be happy that you will end up winning the race in the long term.

<u>What Should Your Diet Look Like When You Want To Burn Fat?</u>

Although the results of different diets can vary from person to person, there are some basic ideas that almost everyone can benefit from.

Remember, unless you are building muscle by lifting weights, you should be trying to lose about 1-2 lbs a week. Keep track of the amount of calories that you usually consume, and then start your diet by consuming about 500 calories less per day.

If you usually consume 3,000 calories a day, you should now be consuming 2,500 calories a day. If you don't lose any weight by the following week, decrease your calories by an additional 250. You would now be consuming 2,250 calories per day.

Continue to decrease your calories by 250 a week until you start to lose weight.

Obviously, there is a limit to how low your calories should go. You should try not to drop below 1,500 calories a day.

Aside from sleep and water, calories are what allow you to function throughout the day. You need calories for energy, and depriving yourself of calories to such an extreme extent can lead to problems.

If you are still not losing weight after consuming only 1,500 calories a day, you might need to increase the amount of time that you spend doing cardiovascular exercise.

Over the years, I've noticed that certain foods seem to work better for losing weight than others. Along with cutting back on calories, you should also be consuming low-calorie foods that will "fill you up" without leaving you feeling extremely hungry an hour later.

Some of the best foods to consume when you are truing to burn fat are:

-Oatmeal
-Fruit
-Egg Whites
-Whole Wheat Bagels
-Boneless, Skinless Chicken
-Brown Rice
-Baked Potatoes without butter or sour cream
-Vegetables
-Low-Fat Yogurt

These foods will give you the necessary calories for energy without interfering with your fat-loss goals. Baked potatoes can be seasoned with salt and pepper in order to avoid any unwanted calories.

Chicken salad can work wonders for fat-loss. Salad alone can leave you feeling hungry, but adding skinless, boneless chicken to it can make a difference.

The meal will still be low in calories, but you will no longer have to worry about being hungry again immediately afterward.

Oatmeal should only cause you to gain weight if you consume it in large enough quantities. Stick with one serving, and then add some egg whites and fruit to the meal for a low-calorie, yet filling breakfast.

You can get as creative as you would like with your diet. You can add olive oil or almonds to your salad.

Chicken doesn't have to be the only type of meat that you consume. There are different kinds of lean meats available, but it's important that you measure everything.

If a certain type of meat is a little bit higher in calories, you will simply need to have less of it.

Stay within your correct calorie range, and try to avoid fattening foods such as pork, butter, whole milk, etc.

Don't forget to allow yourself a couple of meals a week that are not included in your fat-loss diet.

How To Use Beverages To Your Advantage When You Want To Burn Fat

Obviously, you should stay away from soft drinks and other high-sugar beverages when you are trying to burn fat or lose weight, but there are some less obvious things you can do with beverages that can help speed up your fat-burning progress.

Drinking a couple of 8 oz glasses of water right after a meal can really make you feel like you ate a lot more than you actually did.

Drinking too much water at once can make you feel bloated though, so be careful not to overdo it. You can also drink cold water between meals to delay any feelings of hunger that you might have.

Personally, herbal tea has always increased my appetite. It could possibly be due to the fact that herbal tea can be relaxing. I would drink it before bedtime, and then I would have to get out of bed to get a snack. If you notice something similar happening, you might wish to avoid herbal tea.

The type of milk you drink will depend on how much milk you consume. If you drink quite a lot of milk, then it makes sense to stick with the nonfat kind.

If you consume very little milk, you can probably get away with drinking 2% or even whole milk. As always, as long as you stay within your correct calorie range, you should be fine.

A good drink to help you burn fat is vegetable juice. You can either make the juice yourself with the vegetables of your choice, or you can buy the juice that's already made in a container at the store.

The good thing about making the juice at home is that you get to put all the vegetables of your choice into the mix while leaving out all of the vegetables that you really don't care for.

Vegetable juice tends to be thick, and high in vitamins. The thickness can make it feel very filling while the vitamins can help make sure that you aren't deprived of anything that you normally wouldn't be if you were on a high-calorie diet.

Do You Really Need To Eliminate Carbohydrates From Your Diet?

Since each individual is different, it might take some experimentation to find a diet that is right for you.

I have tried many different types of diets that I customized for myself over the years. I experimented with high carbohydrates/low fat, low carbohydrates/high fat, etc. It took some time to clear up the confusion, but I was eventually able to realize that completely eliminating carbohydrates from your diet is not a good idea.

I remember gaining the most fat when I was consuming a high carbohydrate/high fat diet. Losing weight was easy when I switched my diet over to high protein/low fat/low carbohydrates, but I didn't have much energy. I felt tired and hungry most of the time. High fat/low carbohydrates would give me more energy, but it would also leave me feeling hungry.

If you want to burn fat, you cannot be on a diet that consists of high carbohydrates or high fat. It's also important to keep in mind that if you want to have energy, your diet has to have at least some carbohydrates.

A good diet for burning fat should consist of moderate carbohydrates/high protein/low fat. This will ensure that you have enough energy as you burn fat.

Try to consume carbohydrates that are filling. Sugar is known to be considered a carbohydrate, so watch out for that when you are reading food labels. For example, a product might contain 27 grams of carbohydrates per serving.

After you scroll down, you might also see that it contains 23 grams of sugar. That means 23 out of those 27 grams of carbohydrates are actually sugar. Minimizing your sugar intake is important if you wish to burn fat. Stick with brown rice, baked potatoes, and vegetables for your carbohydrate needs. You can even eat pasta as long as you don't exceed your calorie goals.

Since carbohydrates provide you with energy, it makes sense to cut back on them gradually throughout the day. For example, the meal that contains the most carbohydrates should be breakfast.

The meal that contains the least amount of carbohydrates should be your last meal of the day.

Since you are not using a lot of energy when you are asleep, you shouldn't give your body a reason to store the extra carbohydrates that you aren't using as fat.

High-carbohydrate foods are usually cheap, but they can provide a lot of value if you use them correctly. Although I don't believe that you should eliminate the consumption of fat altogether, you should still keep it down to a minimum. It doesn't have to be complicated.

Completely cutting out fat and carbohydrates from your diet is a bit extreme. A well-balanced diet would never call for the elimination of any type of nutrient.

How Often Should You Eat When You Want To Burn Fat?

Many people seem to be under the impression that eating more often will lead to weight gain. They assume that you will have to gain weight if you eat constantly. "Eating constantly" actually sounds really vague.

You need to consider what you're eating, how often you're eating, and how much you are eating.

Gaining weight is not as easy as eating all the time, and losing weight is not as easy as eating less often.

If you eat large meals, your system will feel overloaded. On the other hand, if you don't eat often enough, your body might begin to store fat.

When you only eat a few times a day, you send your body the signal that there is not enough food available. Think about it for a minute.

Let's say that you were getting paid every week at your job. Since you're used to getting a big paycheck every Friday, you don't hesitate to spend your money Saturday through Thursday.

Since you know that your money is going to be replaced, you don't feel like you have to hold onto it.

Now let's say that instead of paying you every week, your employer decides to pay you whenever they feel like it. Sometimes it's once every 3 weeks, and sometimes it's every 5 weeks.

Things start to become uncertain and uncomfortable.

You have a rough time predicting exactly how much money you will need for the entire month, so you start to hold onto the money that you have. You're not exactly sure how you will need your money to last, so you try to play it safe by saving extra cash.

The same thing happens when you don't consume calories regularly. Your body does not know when it's going to get food again, so it tries to store extra fat for emergencies.

Your body is not interested in burning fat when it thinks that there is going to be a shortage of it.

Generally, the more often you eat, the more weight you will lose.

Try not to eat less than 6 times a day when you are trying to burn fat.

It might feel like a chore to have to eat so often, but the good news is that these meals are supposed to be small.

You don't have to turn each meal into a gourmet dinner, but you should make sure that you are eating healthy.

Having a banana with a couple tablespoons of peanut butter can give you about 300 calories without taking up a lot of your time.

Eating every 2 hours will allow you to have 6-8 meals a day. Consuming about 200-300 calories per meal 6-8 times a day will send your body the signal that it doesn't have to worry about not getting enough food.

How often you eat is just as important as what you eat. You want your metabolism to be as fast as possible when you are trying to burn fat.

How To Lift Weights To Burn Fat

Although, I believe that the majority of your fat-loss goals can be achieved mainly through your diet, I also believe that exercise can speed up your progress when you are trying to burn fat.

Exercise will burn extra calories, and if done correctly, can bring shape and definition to the muscles.

Exercise in general will particularly come in handy on those days when you give yourself a "special meal" as a break from your diet.

You learned earlier that having a couple of meals a week that aren't part of your diet can actually be beneficial.

Now you might think, "I won't have to work out if I just skip the pizza and stay on my diet for every single meal for the rest of my life."

Well, you could try to do that, but don't forget that you will be more likely to give up in the long term if you become too rigid with your diet.

Although lifting weights is mainly used for the purpose of building muscle, cardiovascular exercise is not the only type of exercise that burns calories.

You won't burn fat directly through weightlifting, but you will burn calories while you exercise.

Another thing to keep in mind is that, as stated earlier in the book, it's not all about the numbers on a scale.

Although there is no such thing as turning fat into muscle, you can look like you are in much better shape than you really are if you have some quality muscle mass to go along with any extra body fat that you might be carrying.

The idea is to move through your workout fast without sacrificing the use of proper form on the exercises. By moving from exercise to exercise with little to no rest between the sets, you will practically be performing a cardiovascular and weightlifting workout at the same time.

For example, if you are performing a leg workout, you might start with a set of squats. Next, you would immediately do a set of lunges, and then a set of leg curls.

That's three sets in a row without stopping to rest. After doing these three sets, you would rest for a minute before repeating the cycle again.

Instead of doing 3 sets of squats, 3 sets of lunges, and three sets of leg curls, you can simply do one exercise after another as a series, and then repeat the series 3 times.

Another benefit to working out with weights this way is that it saves time.

So it saves time, builds muscle, and burns extra calories.

Talk about productivity!

Is There A Right Or Wrong Way To Do Cardiovascular Exercise?

Burning extra calories is not the only benefit that cardiovascular exercise has to offer. Cardiovascular exercise can also help you feel a lot more flexible.

Carrying around extra body fat can make you feel stiff, and cardiovascular exercise can really help you feel like you are in great shape. If you stay consistent, you can really notice some positive changes in how you feel.

The type of exercises you choose to do are a matter of personal preference. Many people seem to be under the impression that there is a certain exercise that triumphs over the others.

When it comes to weightlifting, there are certain exercises that can help pack on muscle mass faster than others. But when you want to burn fat, the main point of cardiovascular exercise is to burn extra calories.

It's all about doing the things that work best for you. If you don't want to quit after a few weeks, you need to make sure that you are having fun. There are some general rules to follow.

You are working out the wrong way when:

-You dread your next workout session

-You experience intense pain during the workout

-You fail to break a sweat even when the temperature around you is hot

-You feel unusually bored and unmotivated

-You fail to make progress after several months have gone by

-You know that you can do better, but you choose not to try

-You are at a fitness center that fails to meet your needs

Notice how none of these things have anything to do with which exercises you are doing. They also have nothing to do with the time of day that you choose to work out. Take a look at that list and make sure that you are doing everything you can to avoid those things. How you choose to avoid them is up to you.

Some people might choose to stay motivated by watching fitness videos, and others might choose to listen to loud music while they exercise.

Whenever I found something that worked really well, my happiness would increase and I would make better progress as a result.

When someone would say, "You can't do that", I would listen to them, and as a result, my progress would suffer. I finally decided to go back to what my instincts were telling me, and I was not disappointed.

By using happiness and satisfaction as your guide, you can accomplish your goals. You feel happy working out a certain way for a reason, so it's time to start embracing that happiness.

Don't let anyone drag you down by allowing them to convince you to go against your instincts. Feel free to change things around a bit to suit your own personal needs. Gradually change things around until you find something that fits.

Try to aim for about 30-45 minutes of cardiovascular exercise 3-5 times a week. If you are not used to cardiovascular exercise, you will need to work your way up gradually. Start out with just a few minutes every other day if you have to. You don't want to scare yourself away from exercise by doing too much all at once, and then getting a horrible impression of what it's like.

Exercise is very powerful. It can help you or injure you, so it's important that you start slow. Learn to do it the right way in the beginning, and then you can reap the benefits for the rest of your life by staying consistent.

<u>How To Use The Power Of Your Mind To Control Your Body Weight</u>

The body can act as a reflection of the mind.

You need to be in control mentally before you can be in control physically. Thinking positive about life in general is a good thing, but you need to be specific with your thoughts when you are trying to achieve specific goals.

It's important to realize that you can burn fat if you set your mind to it. I know how difficult it is to resist all of the different temptations that present themselves in life.

That's why it's so important to have control over your life, and you take control of your life by not allowing negative, self-defeating thoughts to dwell in your mind.

Even though you give yourself a couple of breaks from your diet every week, you might still find yourself craving food that isn't good for you or your weight-loss goals.

The trick to overcoming these cravings is to simply remember that you will be able to take a break from your diet soon enough.

Oftentimes, we give ourselves the idea that we will never see anything good again. We start a new diet, and then we panic about never being able to be happy again. Instead of feeling liberated from an unhealthy lifestyle, we feel trapped by a healthy lifestyle.

Let's say that your fat-loss diet is strictly followed from Sunday-Friday, and then you have pizza for dinner on Saturday night as a reward. If you get a craving for something that is high in calories on Wednesday, just remember that you only have a few more days to go.

Picture how much better it will be on Saturday night when you can take advantage of a well-deserved break. Remember why you're doing this, and keep your goals in the front of your mind at all times.

Don't give in.

The negative feelings involved with regret usually outweigh any feelings that come along with self-indulgence.

When you're unsure of what you should do, just ask yourself, "Will this bring me closer to my fat-loss goals?"

Make sure that you fully appreciate what you are doing. Every workout counts, and each day that you stick to your diet counts as another step toward a new and better life.

Your hard work will pay off, but you have to stay consistent. It's much easier to stay consistent when you have something to look forward to.

Far too many people tend to get discouraged when they don't see the results they're looking for right away. Don't worry about making mistakes.

There will be days when you lose your motivation, but it always finds its way back. As long as you don't allow the short- term setbacks to stop you from realizing your fat-loss dreams, you can win in the long term.

Judging your progress based on what has happened over the course of a few weeks will not always give you an accurate indication of where you're at. Sometimes you have to wait a few years before you can truly appreciate just how far you have really come with your goals.

The truth is that we are usually making progress every day, but it can be difficult to see it before a substantial amount of time has passed by. It's similar to growing in height when you are a kid.

You don't notice yourself getting taller by the day, so you get impatient. It starts to feel as if you will never get taller.

But when you grow 7 inches after a few years, you begin to realize that you were actually growing all along.

Most people will look at supplements as an easy solution. What they don't seem to realize is that supplements will not help you if your mind is not in the right place.

Once you have the right mindset, supplements become less important.

Everything you need to achieve your fat-loss goals will just seem to come along naturally.

You should never feel discouraged when something is taking a long time to happen.

Usually, the best things in life will require the most time and dedication. But that's how you will know that they are worthy of pursuing.

Your body weight might bounce back and forth as you try to burn fat. This used to happen to me all the time.

The important thing to remember is that it's just one step back in order to take a couple of steps forward. Taking shortcuts will make you more likely to gain back the fat, so try to stay patient.

Once you achieve a new, healthy lifestyle, it will be easier to stay consistent with your diet, workout plan, etc. You just need to take that first step.

It gets easier after you start seeing the results. After you look in the mirror to see your how much your hard work paid off, you will know that it has been worth it.